# A Growing Faith

## Stories from Bed

# Praise for A Growing Faith

"*A Growing Faith* is a brief look into the life of someone who has suffered from this horrible, insidious condition known as RSD or CRPS. It is less a medical primer and more a how-to on dealing with chronic pain and other symptoms with faith and a positive outlook. A rare and precious gem!"

Mike and Sandra Worley
Yuma, AZ

"*A Growing Faith* is a heart wrenching, yet uplifting journal of her battle with the disabling disease RSD. She is filled with courage, faith and resilience. She stays positive at some of the most trying times in her life."

Heather Wilda, Teacher with RSD
Concordia Charter School, Chandler, AZ

"*A Growing Faith* is an inspiration to all who read it. It lets every person that suffers with RSDS/CRPS know that life is a journey and with support from family and friends they can make it. With the advancement in Research a cure will come."

Dorothy Cormier, Caregiver
Cornerstone Community Health Services

# A Growing Faith

## Stories from Bed

MARY JANE GONZALES

TATE PUBLISHING
AND ENTERPRISES, LLC

*A Growing Faith*


Published by Tate Publishing & Enterprises, LLC
127 E. Trade Center Terrace | Mustang, Oklahoma 73064 USA
1.888.361.9473 | www.tatepublishing.com

Tate Publishing is committed to excellence in the publishing industry. The company reflects the philosophy established by the founders, based on Psalm 68:11,
*"The Lord gave the word and great was the company of those who published it."*


*Cover design by Jan Sunday Quilaquil*
*Interior design by Joana Quilantang*

Published in the United States of America

ISBN: 978-1-62295-925-9
1. Biography & Autobiography / Personal Memoirs
2. Medical / Diseases
12.12.03

# Dedication

This book is dedicated to those with RSDS/CRPS and chronic pain sufferers everywhere, to the patients and advocates, their families and friends, and everyone working toward awareness and a cure.

# Acknowledgment

I would like to acknowledge my partner in pain, Heather Wilda. Heather and I met through the mentoring program offered by RSD Hope. Heather is new to RSD, yet has become full-body in less than two years. Despite the pain and difficulty she goes through, she is very level-headed. She does her research, seeks appropriate treatment and has a positive attitude. Thank you, Heather, for your friendship and your tips to clarify certain things within this book. As I continue to write and share, it's people like you who make it all worthwhile.

# Contents

# Preface

Since the writing of my book In the Blink of an Eye... My Life with RSDS, my condition has changed dramatically. This journal/blog book is my continuing story and my attempt at raising public awareness of RSDS/CRPS, a debilitating disease/condition, for which there is no cure. We in the RSDS community are seeking research in hope of a cure.

# Culture Shock

In the marketing stage of the first book, I sent out letters to RSDS support groups to announce the book, and some people responded back, which led to new friendships or acquaintances. This was great, of course, but it was also like culture shock because suddenly I was interacting with people who understood my disease/situation. There were so many stories, with both commonalities and differences. I was amazed at the number of people who were crusaders for the cause through blogs, websites, events, etc. I kind of felt guilty that I had waited so long to get involved, that I had not acted sooner, that I had been an island unto myself, so to speak.

Now I'm seeing this vast movement of people, rallying together for the cause. The numbers are astonishing and there's strength in numbers so, no doubt, there will be great effect. I have such hope for strides in research, leading to treatment and a possible cure. Though, at the same time, I have great sorrow that it may come too late for me. I have an e-mail friend who went to the hospital this weekend in an ambulance and was shocked that none of the ambulance crew had ever heard of RSD and later, at the hospital, only one person had heard of it. Because not much is known about the disease, those affected by it are subjected to standard protocol which could jeopardize them severely. Yet, in the same week, news broke that "researchers have identified a gene related to chronic pain; thereby, signaling a significant step toward better understanding and treating of the condition." What exciting news that is!

# My Friend with RSD

One of my closest friends hurt her foot two years ago. She has suffered intense pain and was recently diagnosed with RSD. The diagnosis came as no surprise because her symptoms were identical to mine. Her pain was so bad that the doctor had her on morphine until recently, when she went to an acupuncturist and it took away all her pain. She does quite well with the acupuncture as long as she goes three times a week, but if she misses a treatment she will relapse. Apparently, it's like everything else out there: a band-aid, not a cure. But to be fair, she hasn't been going very long. Time will tell if a cure is on the horizon. Yet, even without a cure, relief is welcome.

Ironically, I had gone to an acupuncturist years ago but, when he discovered I was also seeing a chiropractor, he stopped treating me. He said he wouldn't treat me if I was seeing someone else, because when I get healed he can't take the credit for it. Since I would not give up my chiropractor, who I had been seeing for probably a decade, I forfeited the chance at acupuncture. I hate that it worked out that way but I do understand his point. Eventually even the chiropractor stopped treating me because I was too frail. He said I had the body of a ninety-year-old woman, and that was like twenty years ago.

# Shoulder Injuries

The new injuries I referred to in the first chapter are injuries to the shoulders. Note that is plural. The left shoulder got injured first when I was stripping the bed. I tugged at the sheet and suddenly pain exploded in my shoulder, which radiated down my arm, encompassing the elbow and hand. That limb is so vital to me maneuvering in and out of bed as I have to scoot across the bed on that elbow in order to get up. So now much of that movement involves crying or screaming out in pain. Using my right side for that is not an option, as my right side is even more limited than the left side. And, because of the "mirror image" factor, my right shoulder has now been injured just by reaching for something. Needless to say, life has become far more challenging and faith is needed more than ever. I know not everyone believes in God and I know to them I may sound fanatical, but I know He is real by what He has done inside me. I often wonder…if pain and debilitation are so hard for me, a believer who leans on and trusts in a mighty God, how on earth does an unbeliever cope? Who do they lean on and trust in that is big enough or capable to affect their situation? Where do they get the strength to overcome trials and sorrow?

prayer that I would walk in sweet fellowship and submission to God.

I believe there are no super Christians, just ordinary people called or expected to do extraordinary things (like losing a loved one, living with disease, etc.). I can only pray (figuratively) that each time I fall down I will get right back up and, too, that I will finish well.

# Working Toward Change

Most all the people I've met who have RSDS are speaking out about it and working toward change. One woman has a website, a blog and a support group. Another woman has a wellness store, a website and a support group. Yet another has yard sales to benefit the RSDSA. The internet is loaded with blogs and websites related to RSDS. So, the classification of rare disease is not from the number of people affected by it. Rather, it is because so little is known about it. This past weekend (Labor Day 2010) was the Muscular Dystrophy telethon and Jerry Lewis was saying that forty-five years ago, when they first started out, the chance of a cure was very slim. Now the chance of a cure is very good. Imagine what feelings of hope that stirred in me (and every other person with a debilitating disease) as it means there is hope of a cure for RSDS!

# Leg Ulcers

In this heightened state with the new shoulder injuries, I have also had leg ulcers for six out of ten months. Leg ulcers are dangerous and painful and require wound care treatment. In my case, poor circulation causes body fluids to seep out the pores, which leads to ulcers, but with or without ulcers the moisture from the weeping creates fungus (which is neither fun nor easy to deal with). When cleaning the ulcers and/or fungus, the wash cloths can't be re-used, so that can be quite costly, buying wash cloths each week only to use them once and throw them away. Plus, linens need laundering every day from the weeping. That, too, is costly if you use commercial machines.

With regard to the shoulder, it may have a torn rotator cuff in addition to RSDS, but, since I am not a candidate for surgery, we're not pursuing it. i.e. Surgery is risky as it can cause RSDS, spread RSDS or worsen RSDS; and, with my extreme frailty, there would be an even greater risk.

With regard to venous stasis ulcers, I have had them yet again and worse than ever. From the end of my toes to the mid shin was one big oozing, bleeding mess that became one gigantic scab, which landed me in bed 24/7. Sadly, this was the fault of my nurse who saw the ulcers coming back and wouldn't increase my visits/care. When my condition got this bad as a result of her neglect, we talked about it and she admitted her wrong but did not apologize. I had been very fond of her, but jeopardizing my health like this was too much for me to bear, not just painwise, but more so robbing me of my independence. However limited it had been, I treasured the ability to get around my apartment for things I needed, and now that was lost to me. It remains to be seen whether or not I will walk again. It doesn't look good, but faith and determination are powerful forces to which I cling. Regarding the nurse and what had transpired, I decided to let her go. So I changed agencies and ended up with someone better who was far more gentle and came every day, rain or shine. Another contention for me with the old nursing agency was the standard treatment called "Debriding" which means to remove the old tissue from the wound area. I think it is usually scraped off with a scalpel but, with me being so frail, it was rubbed off briskly and forcibly with a cloth, which was still very painful, though, certainly, not as painful as using a tool. It was then followed up with a "Wet to dry" wrap, but the gauze would adhere to the moisture of my weeping legs and feet. Then, upon drying, it would be torture to remove the gauze and usually made matters worse. So I came away from that experience with a fierce determination to take charge of my own care and well-being, meaning that I would not sit back and let people dictate to me what would or wouldn't be done concerning my care. So with the new agency I specified what I wanted, based on the uniqueness of my body, i.e. frailty and special needs. With my doctor's consent, the new nursing agency agreed to try this unorthodox treatment plan, which worked out wonderfully for me. It still involved cleaning the wound and rubbing to remove old tissue (but with less pressure) and never covering the wound. That way there was no sticking of gauze and no tearing of tissue upon removing the gauze. Saline was used to cleanse and heal the ulcers by drying them out. The ulcers, though (being so bad), required total bed rest and took nearly two months to heal enough for me to even attempt sitting up. Because of the many disabilities (particularly the shoulder), the now healed ulcers were just the start of the road to recovery, as my body had weakened over two months and I had to begin the journey back with only fifteen minutes of "sitting up" per day, increasing it a little more each week. When combined with the shoulder injury, I am not yet able to sit up on my own, though I'm determined to get there. And even if I manage (at some point) to do that, the next step would be "getting up." All of this is a lengthy process and a scary one in light of my limitations, but my faith in God sees me through. Although I am still in bed, I have no complaints of discomfort or discontent, which I find amazing. In addition to that, He has…at the worst time of my life, given me the best care possible. A skilled and caring provider, a close friend who came and stayed with me for several days at the height of the pain when I could do hardly anything for myself. Plus, a friend who took over my grocery shopping to help out the caregiver, as well as assistance from neighbors who let me call them day or night, who ran errands and cooked meals. More stories of grace, just like the first book. I am also amazed that a wound that size did not scar one iota. Kudos to my doctor, who works with me, adapting to my special needs, and a nurse who does likewise. I am so blessed!...And if telling my story can help someone else, that would be an added blessing!

# More Impaired

On this journey of restoration, although I am intent on sitting up every day and regaining strength, sometimes I get hurt in the process and there are times when those new injuries prevent me from doing so; like today…a hip injury, and last week…a hand injury. It's disappointing because it causes me to lose momentum, but I can't dwell on it. I have to be tenacious in my pursuit. And I need people close to me to "go with the flow" by moving on when possible and holding back when necessary. Whether it's a nurse, caregiver, friend or family member, they need to trust/believe me, not judge me. If they don't trust/believe me, their perception will hurt and hinder me. Common perceptions of people unrelated to the medical field are: thinking I'm lazy, that I don't try hard enough, I'm a drama queen/attention seeker, etc. These attitudes are toxic and may need to be weeded out of your life. Surround yourself with supportive, nurturing types. It adds so much to your quality of life.

Well, it is now weeks later and I have had a barrage of injuries from trying to sit up, each worse than the last, that have all lingered. It's pretty discouraging. And my toes are falling more and more each day, a condition called drop foot, where you lose muscle, the foot becomes rigid and starts to fall. (Also discouraging.) Yesterday I cried because it's looking more and more like this might be permanent. That doesn't mean I've given up hope. It just means that I have to consider this might be the will of God, for a particular purpose or plan. As much as I dislike that thought, I'm trying to be yielded.

Here I am again, weeks later still. Not only have I not healed from the injuries I incurred while trying each day to sit up, the accumulation of injuries to the shoulder, back and buttocks have rendered me more impaired. Plus, my shoulder and hip have become concave; meaning atrophied (which prevents me from even trying to sit up). I am beside myself! How does one explain (or live) a total trust in God despite feeling the weight and heaviness of despair? How does one abide with the almighty when everything dear and vital to them has been stripped away? I started to say "I don't know." Then I realized that actually I do know. I'm referring to the love…the love that surpasses any I have ever known, a love that is truly unconditional and cares and provides for me better than any other ever has, strong enough to give "peace that passes all understanding" and "calm amidst the storm."

If I couldn't abide in the Lord, I would have total despair and darkness.

# Part Two

I started a blog recently, hoping to help and effect others with RSD, hoping to raise public awareness as well. I try to write in it only when I feel inspired of God, instead of my natural ramblings. I recently wrote a song about my journey with RSD and it has been put to music. I heard it sung today for the first time and it brought me to tears. I pray that God will expedite the full recording of it so I can share it with the RSD community. The world of chronic pain sufferers is increasingly vast and it's important for everyone to tell their story for the sake of awareness and research. So, herein, is Part Two of my story. Why do I call it A Growing Faith? Because the less able I become, the more obvious His provision is. I could go on but that's the bottom line.

At present, I am still in bed, unable to get up on my own and too frail to be lifted by a person or a device. Since being in bed, I have found it very hard to read lying down, although I am able to craft lying down. Who knew?! Lastly, believing there is a divine purpose in this, how can I complain about my suffering to the Lord Jesus Christ, knowing all that He suffered for me?

# New to Blogging

Though new to the world of blogging, I am not new to the world of RSDS/CRPS. I have had RSD for approximately twenty-six years and wasn't diagnosed until eight years ago. Chiropractic, acupuncture and a brief attempt at PT were no match for this debilitating disease. By the time I was diagnosed, RSD had consumed my body and left me homebound. Like so many others, I know what it's like to be told repeatedly by doctors "I can't help you because I don't know what 's wrong." Before the diagnosis, some people thought I was faking or exaggerating but that pretty much changed after the diagnosis, except that there will always be some who don't get it. I am blessed to have a good support system among family and friends, and I pray the same for all RSD-ers. When I was first diagnosed I was helped tremendously by Linda Lang's book Living with RSDS and it is my hope that my book In the Blink of an Eye will likewise help others. Blessings to all RSD-ers. May you find relief, if not healing.

# Here I Am Again

Here I am again, doing something I never thought I would do, as I'm totally clueless about blogs...but I was recently inspired by my eleven-year-old granddaughter who started one and I knew if she could do it, so could I. First of all, I need to state the name of our disease. Previously, I used the initials RSDS/CRPS, which stands for Reflex Sympathetic Dystrophy Syndrome (newly named Chronic Regional Pain Syndrome). Throughout the blog, I will generally refer to the disease as RSD. Secondly, I need to state that I am not a clinician, just a long-time patient, speaking from experience. RSD is a neurological condition that effects nerves, joints and tissue. Injuries travel to (and settle in) the nearest joint, nerve pain creates intense burning, and skin is tissue...which explains why it hurts for people to touch us. I've heard from some that it also affects bone but I have not experienced that. The pain and symptoms we incur are way disproportionate to the actual injury and linger long after the injury should be healed. The reason for this is that messages are not getting through between the nervous system and the brain, telling it how much to hurt and when to stop hurting. It's basically a short circuit in the nervous system. The analogy I often use is that of a car alarm. When working properly, it is intended to alert you of a break-in but, when not working properly, it goes haywire, beeping incessantly from invalid causes such as someone just walking by. While I'm trying to be explicit, I want to keep it simple. Hopefully, I can find the right balance. So consider that kind of pain and factor in disbelief from people in your life. Though the symptoms are bizarre and the pain is unbelievable, what's needed more than understanding is trust, trust that the patient wouldn't lie or exaggerate their symptoms. Otherwise, you could end up with a strained relationship that would cause you both to suffer and cause the patient to be isolated. On the flip side, where there's trust or unconditional love, the patient receives needed support and your union with them is enhanced. I sincerely hope this blog will be of help to you in some way or other.

Blessings.
Jane

# The Question Of Touch

I have been asked four times in the last two weeks why I tell people "Don't touch me." and, yet, some people do/ need to touch me. "What is the difference?" they ask. "Why can those people (nurse, doctor, caregiver) touch you, but not others?" Well...it's a good question to ask but a difficult one to answer. I will try to explain it as best I can, bearing in mind I don't fully understand it either. These are the things of which I am cognizant that would understandably make a difference.

First of all, because of the risk, there would have to be a need. For example: the nurse may need to do wound care treatment. So she would jokingly say "Assume the position." Then I would position myself for her to treat my feet and legs. Next, I would brace myself by clinching the sheet tightly (with both hands) to bear the touch. Like driving down the road, if your car hits a big bump or a pothole that jolts your body, it could hurt or misalign you. Whereas, if you knew it was up ahead, you would brace yourself for it and not be hurt. Gone are the days of hugging people. No matter how much I said "gentle," I would still get hurt. So now I get "virtual hugs" from friends and kisses from family. I realize I am super frail and being gentle is critical for any touch. Whether or not this is representative of other

RSDers, I don't know. I have often wondered about that and would welcome any and all responses, to get an assessment of that. Blessings to all who suffer with this disease and blessings to those who desire to understand,

Jane

# A Song In The Making ("My Only Consolation")

My poem about RSD has just been put to music and will soon be recorded, God willing.

I've had this thing forever
This thing called RSD
No matter where or when,
It kept pursuing me
One place, then another,
It never would relent
Attacking all my body parts
Until they all were spent
I fought my best to beat it
Never giving in
The fiercest pain I'd ever known
Was pushing hard to win
All the years I battled
To keep this thing at bay
But in the end, seemingly,

I didn't have a say
My only consolation
And comfort through it all
Is knowing I was not alone,
My God was standing tall
Standing right beside me
And holding tight my hand
Whispering "I love you"
And "I have got a plan"
"A plan for good and not for bad
But you will have to trust
That this is meant to strengthen you
Although it seems unjust"

# Gratitude

Greetings, everyone! I hope those of you with RSD are having a low-pain day. There's something I've been meaning to write about for a long time but, not knowing how to express it, I had put it on the back burner, so to speak. Thus, it is long overdue and I can't procrastinate anymore. The subject is gratitude. In this world, we can be so consumed with problems or busyness that we lose sight of or take things for granted. We sometimes miss the good because we're blinded by the bad. And yet there's so much good all around us. I am grateful for the medicine I take for pain relief; though it doesn't heal me, it makes things bearable. I'm grateful for a caring, compassionate doctor (who makes house calls) and good caregivers. And I'm thankful for you…the friends and family who help and support me; who share with me, laugh with me, cry with me, counsel me and just plain care. God has blessed me with very special people and I want you all to know how much you're appreciated. With love and hugs, Jane

# A Song Completed

I'm so excited to share with you that the song I posted on here back in April ("My Only Consolation") has now been put to music by a very talented singer/songwriter, Lequita Hoffpauir. God has blessed this endeavor and to Him be the glory. My hope is for it to be sold online at Amazon, iTunes and CD Baby.

# A Secret Revealed

The spring issue of the RSDSA newsletter was jolting to me as I read about the secret Linda Lang has been keeping; that she has been mostly bed bound for the last eighteen months. I have been a huge fan of Linda ever since I read her book eight years ago. Though we never met, she's been a mentor of sorts through her book and all she imparts. For that reason, my heart went out to her that she was in a worsened state, as I feel akin to her somehow. Plus, reading the article about her secret was very convicting to me , as I have been keeping a secret of the same nature. You see, I have been homebound for years and bed bound (loosely speaking), as my bed was the only place I could access with my physical limitations. So that space became my whole little world, which I talked about in my book In the Blink of an Eye. But eight months ago, I developed severe leg ulcers and was confined to bed, lying down. About six weeks in, I started sitting up a few minutes each day. Rather, I should say tried sitting up each day. The reality is I sometimes made it and sometimes didn't, but either way, the attempts would injure me time and time again, resulting in more disabilities that ultimately prevented me from getting up at all, including muscle atrophy, which solidified things. So this was my secret ...that I was now truly, totally bed bound. I could say honestly to my friends that I was writing a new book and I didn't want people to know what was in the second book before reading the first book. However, what I didn't tell them was that I was embarrassed or ashamed to be so limited and so needy. I didn't want to be pitied or shunned. But Linda's article really did convict me that we're a community and we need to be there for each other, with moral support, prayer support and all else. For myself, it convicted me too that instead of focusing on being bed bound, I need to focus on the fact that it took twenty-six years to get this way. With all that I've been through, I'm glad that my body lasted as long as it did and I'm glad that RSD is now being diagnosed earlier than before so that some people are now experiencing relief or improvement with early treatment. We all need to share our stories and respect each other's situation with the understanding that, despite all the commonalities, RSD affects everyone differently. We need to pray for each other, sharing each other's victories and mourning each other's losses. And, above all else, we need to pray for a cure...that no more people, especially children, would have to endure such pain and debilitation.

# I Have Concluded

I love my life! …most of it, anyway. Do I want to be bed bound? No. But is it without redemption? No. While it's true that I live with horrendous pain and debilitation, confinement and related issues, it is also true that I have a life. I may not be able-bodied any longer but I'm still able…. able to live at home, able to have adequate care, able to do hobbies, able to function in my own little corner of the world. Am I seeing through rose-colored glasses? No. I see the bad and I cope with it every day, but it's not my focus. Rather than being consumed by despair, I want to be cognizant of grace. Just as Joseph Aquilino found his entrepreneurial "gift" through RSD by hosting radio shows and advocating for many causes, I found the spirit within that fights to overcome every trial, the "stretching" of God to meet every challenge, and provision of God to meet every need. Yet, though I would like to be content in any situation, admittedly it has taken nine months to acclimate to the latest upheaval. Like not being able to access my 12" computer, needing instead to use an 8.9" netbook that I can prop up against my arm sideways (which is indeed a blessing but I'm still missing the greeting card software on the 12"), learning to craft upside down but being unable to read books or magazines upside down, spending a fortune on disposable items like paper plates, paper cups, hand wipes, plastic bags, etc., positioning everything within my reach and, most of all, emotional acceptance of this lifestyle. Through twenty-six years of RSD, there have been many levels of adjustment and this has been the hardest, but finally I could form and process my thoughts, seeing the reality that life goes on. Thus, I appreciate my family and friends who stand by me, who encourage, help and inspire me. They bless me richly. I hope this post won't sound "Pollyannaish." I just believe that choosing to be positive in a negative circumstance is survival of the fittest.

God bless all RSD'ers, no matter their age or station in life…young or old, married or single. May our efforts at raising awareness truly expedite a cure for RSD.

# A Charmed Life

Although this post is not about RSD, that's ok because RSD is not the sum of me , just a part of me. This post is about my memories of growing up in a small town... Though young at heart, I am a senior citizen (older than dirt, haha). Despite growing up in a dysfunctional home, I have great memories of growing up in New England: ice skating at the park, roller skating down the hill where we lived, the candy store and ice cream parlor nearby, four seasons, foliage and snow. Our home in Reading, MA, was a big two-story house with lots of charm and lots of hiding places. It had two attics, two basements and two long porches, a banister to slide down and a hidden stairway that had been cut off (becoming yet another hiding place). I remember boy friends and best friends and the local movie theater which cost twenty-five cents for the matinee. I remember climbing out my bedroom window and playing dolls on the roof of the front porch. Although, my favorite memory is of the wintertime, as we lived on a hill and the side of the house had a rock wall extending from the back porch down to the back yard. Add to that the height of the porch railing and now you have a good distance, ideal for jumping off the railing into the snow mounds below. Though this account does not detail the antics of a mischievous child (like skipping school, sneaking out at night, etc.), those too are cherished memories. Apart from the tumult of a dysfunctional home, the setting where I grew up was similar to a Norman Rockwell painting. It was the 1950's and 60's in a suburb of Boston. My dad worked for (and later owned) the town cab company, my mother worked at the town diner and we would ride the train into Boston to attend Red Sox games. We were big fans, especially of Ted Williams and the like. Now those were the days. My older brother and I were close in age, so he would get crushes on my friends and I would get crushes on his friends. The bowling alley was the local hangout, as was the drive-in movie theater. They were simpler times back then that evolved into fond memories. Roots grow deep and love endures. We may stray at times but family is forever and I'm glad that my siblings and I are close knit.

It's funny how even little things can leave a big impression, things as simple as doing the dishes. That's where I learned all the secrets typically kept from children... like Santa Claus is not real, there is no Easter bunny, and Mommy was married to someone else before Daddy. What? Yup! She eloped as a teenager and Grandpa had it annulled. Oh, my gosh! No wonder I was a tattle-tale. It probably stemmed from all the times of saying "Mommy! Nickie just said................!" And the baby (the favored one), however cute, was not welcomed to tag along with me (the big sister) as it interrupted my fun. Good thing roots grow deep and love endures.

In my pre-school days, I would have tea parties with my best friend in a wonderful playhouse that was built by her dad. We used to have such fun…until my family moved away when I was six. I missed her terribly but life was too busy to visit back and forth across town, as my mother worked two or three jobs to support us. My mother was very domestic and made all my clothes. Plus, despite working so much, there was always a plate of home-made cookies awaiting us when we arrived home from school. To this day, my childhood friends remember that fondly.

In elementary school, I met my next best friend and we were inseparable. They had a huge house and I would sleep over a lot. I even lived with them a few times. Their family kind of adopted me and I came to be called "the fifth sister." We would pick fruit from their orchard and vegetables from their garden. We carried fresh tomatoes with us everywhere we went, even a salt shaker. We would make pot holders and sell them to earn money for Christmas shopping. We even ran away together once.

In high school, I had another best friend and more excitement. She, too, was very special and we had lots of fun together. Even in adulthood, I wouldn't dream of going home without visiting her. The friends I grew up with were remarkable then and they're remarkable now. I always felt that growing up in Reading was "a charmed life" and, even though so much has changed over the years, I know from my former classmates who still live there that it has remained an ideal community.

# Encouragement

Although writing about RSD is easy because you live it and, therefore, know it…writing about it can also be hard in the sense of distinguishing between the difficulties and the blessings. What blessings, you ask! Many! Like perseverance/tenacity, that determination and fighting spirit that pushes you on, against all odds. You may be battling pain only, you may be battling pain and limitations, or you may reach an impasse, whereby certain body parts that limited movement before, now prevent movement. Regardless of the place you're at, it's your body, not your mind, that is being diminished. You are still you, albeit functioning differently. Like the saying "If Plan A doesn't work, switch to Plan B." For me, doing that gives purpose; it keeps me from stagnating and it keeps me from sinking. So, without meaning to minimize the loss of our normal life, the passions and abilities we discover within our alternate life are the blessings to which I'm referring.

Those of us with RSD are in the fight of our life, trying to survive the pain and hold onto whatever abilities we have. I, for one, have learned that I took things for granted. I assumed I would always be able to walk or brush my hair, or…(fill in the blanks). And I have learned how to make lemonade…haha! A very important life lesson that sometimes involves "searching" for good, as opposed to "seeing" good. This takes daily practice, and it doesn't mean someone is oblivious to their suffering. It means they choose to rise above it…and probably more for the sake of survival than for excellence.

Having persevered for twenty-six years with RSD, I try to encourage others with the disease but I need to encourage myself, as well, as I can't give what I don't have. I find my encouragement in the Word of God and in the person of Jesus Christ. I don't say all this to preach to anyone. I say it to offer hope and encouragement to those who are hurting, that you would know there is a strength greater than your own—just for the asking. There is hope for healing and the promise of sustenance. There is love unconditional and life eternal. Christianity is a relationship, not a religion. "Trust in the Lord with all your heart and lean not on your own understanding; In all your ways acknowledge Him, and He will make your paths straight." Proverbs 3:5-6 NIV. "Taste and see that the Lord is good; blessed is the man who takes refuge in Him." Psalm 34:8 NIV. This was meant to edify, and I sincerely hope that it ministered to someone.

Blessings,
Jane

# A Week of Poetry

I thought I would share some poems that stem from RSD. Though most of them end on a positive note, some of them begin with great despair. So I will play it safe by starting-with inspirational ones rather than dark ones. (One a day for a week)

# It's Important

God it's so important here that you be glorified
As you count all of the agonizing tears that I have cried
It's important God to know I've not run the race in vain
As I wearily endured such a heavy load of pain
It's important in this tunnel God to see light at the end
It's important for the world to see that you're my closest friend
It's important that they know Lord despite my stinky flesh
You and I are in communion and with you I try to mesh
It's important that my witness not relate to sin of man
But in greater part to you as they see your outstretched hand

# Strengthening My Frame

Father God I pray
That you would help me with my feet
That you'd get me safe to bed
And you'd grant me restful sleep
That you'd take away the swelling
And diminish all the pain
That you'd soon begin the process Lord
Of strengthening my frame
That your grace would still continue
In a multitude of ways
And that you would soon incorporate
Healing to my days
Lord I've had to lean upon you
In a state of total need
And while staying by your side
I desire to be freed
From the bondage of dependence
That is burdening my friends
To a relative remission
That on God alone depends
Lord it's not that I'm ungrateful
I see all that you have done
I'm just longing to go forward
That captivity be undone

# Setbacks

God I truly thank you
That it wasn't any worse
But I feel as if my body's been
Attacked by Satan's curse
Every day holds a new injury
Or a problem of some sort
When talking with my friends
I'm embarrassed to report
The ups and downs, the back and forth
The setbacks that occur
Frustration I experience
When healing is deferred

# Move Upon Me, Lord

Father God I pray that you would get me through this time
That your spirit move upon me Lord with laughter and with rhyme
That the ashes turn to beauty and the weeping turn to joy
That the world would see the blessings and the help that you employ
That your grace would be sufficient and your mercies new each day
That when undergoing trials you would teach me how to pray
You would teach me how to worship and commit to you each day
All the things that I hold onto Lord no matter what I say
That my eyes would not be blinded...that the scales would be removed
That you'd strengthen me in spirit and my heart would be renewed

# Rock of Ages

Father, I am sinking
Would you throw to me a rope
Would you please confirm the scripture
That I'm never without hope
Would you strengthen me in spirit
As I trod this rocky road
Would you bear for me the burden
That is such a heavy load
Would you wipe away the tears
That keep falling from my eyes
Would you lovingly send mercy
When you hear my anguished cries
Would you not let pain consume me
Taking focus out of prayer
Would you be my Rock of Ages
Greater than my worldly care

This poem is the stinging reality of life with RSD. Tomorrow I will end the Week of Poetry on a more positive note but, for now, this is the story that needs to be told...this is the awareness that needs to be raised.

# Glimpses of Your Love

In the ravages of illness
In the sorrow and despair
I see glimpses of your love for me
And evidence of care
For despite the tribulation
You are always by my side
In the furnace of affliction
And the many tears I cry
Lord, your grace is so sufficient
Meeting needs of every kind
Paying bills without an income
Causing hearts to re-align
Forming something out of nothing
Making ordinary great
And producing such a witness
From a seeming hopeless fate
Lord, I marvel at your wonders
And your heart that loves me so
Lord, through blessing or through trial
May my praise forever flow

# RSD Awareness Month 2011

Well, here it is November first and the message I've been planning to post was somehow incomplete. I've been planning it for a week but there was something missing and I didn't know what. I only knew I couldn't post until it came to me. What I did know I wanted to write about was a combination of emotions that November holds for me. First, I guess, is the stark reality and sorrow that comes with having RSD. What more can I say? Anyone with RSD knows that no further explanation is needed. I know we're a long way from finding a cure but, on the brighter side, we've come along way; long enough to have LOTS of blogs, websites and research on RSD/CRPS...long enough to even have an "RSD Awareness Month". For me, having had RSD for nearly twenty-seven years, having an awareness month is huge! Also in the mix of emotions is gratitude. In the spirit of Thanksgiving (another November awareness day), I am thankful in this "alternate life" of pain and debilitation, for the ability to re-invent myself through God's grace and find contentment in Him. Lastly, the part that I knew was missing and important enough to hold up the post came to me as I read today's e-mail from American Pain Foundation. I truly don't mean to copy their message; rather, to personalize it. Though we all have friends, chronic pain sufferers can lose a lot of friends from being too needy/burdensome or lack of understanding that equates to disbelief. Thus, we have much appreciation for those who remain close to us. And, yet, there are those who go above and beyond; giving and doing things that are beyond belief...the unsung heroes in our lives. This thought really struck me when I read the e-mail from APF as I am so honored and blessed by unsung heroes...and I pray that you are, too. Though November holds more RSD emotions for me, I will save those for my visit with Joseph Aquilino on his BlogTalkRadio show "The Positive Experience" November 10th at 7 p.m.EST .

# RSD Awareness Month

In November as always
You see us come forth
Sharing our stories,
Discussing our course
The toll of disease
The public must hear
To expedite research
Ensuring a cure
Of CRPS/RSD
And it's dire effects upon you and me
Help us unite, God, in spreading the word
And strengthen our voices
That we would be heard
Help us to educate
Those who don't know
And teach us endurance
As we travel this road

# The Holidays and A Message of Hope

As Thanksgiving approaches, I am thankful for the people in my life and the opportunities that God affords me. I am thankful for all the stories and all the stats and all the heightened advocacy in this month of RSD Awareness. I'm glad to have a sense of community and a hope that we're making a difference in this crusade. May we all have a good Thanksgiving, a good support system and a genuine awareness of God's great love for us.

With this being RSD Awareness Month, I would very much like to offer a message of hope to chronic pain sufferers through a homemade Christmas card. Anyone wishing to receive a card can send their address to mgonzales182@comcast.net Christmas is my favorite time of the year and I look forward to this but, due to finances, I can only send a card to 100 people.

# RSD-A Mystery

There is so much about RSD that doesn't make sense to me. Of course that refers to the disease itself, the misfirings, the frailty, the inadequate treatments and futility regarding a cure. But, on a personal note, my own current condition is baffling to me. I've read numerous times that the symptoms settle down at some point, and I have found that to be true. After twenty plus years, the burning associated with older injuries has subsided...which is a tremendous relief. But it doesn't negate or reverse the disabilities resulting from those injuries...denoting, to me, relief–not remission. And don't be misled...the frailty is ever-present, subjecting me to new injuries.

Though one would assume the patient is now on "easy street" from the relief, that's not really true because, ironically, that's when the secondary symptoms occur. You know, the vision, the vertigo, the unbelievable acid reflux, the trouble swallowing, etc. Who knew the level of pain or discomfort they could cause? I surely didn't. Again, please don't be misled. I am still grateful for the blessings and grace in my life, but I was unprepared for this turn of events. Nor was I prepared for becoming bed bound, which happened a year ago this past week. By the grace of God, I can still function in this alternate life and seem to be busier than ever in this battle for my life and the crusade for awareness. One could even say it's become an obsession for me. As November comes to a close, let us not lose momentum in our drive and our efforts. Let the strength in numbers intensify our voice, that the world would hear and respond.

# The Christmas Season

I'm trying my best to make RSD
Be dormant this Christmas, or better yet flee
I'm trying my best to lay it aside
And focus on Jesus, my Savior and Guide
The reason for joy in the depths of my soul
Despite being broken, He makes me feel whole
He makes me complete in the core of my being
As through Him, it's truth and love I am seeing

In this month of December, my time will be devoted to a Christmas blog, to celebrate the birth of our Lord and Savior, Jesus Christ. Please visit my other blog...A Christmas Collection...and rejoice with me in the gift of His presence.

# They Don't "See Us"

Although I didn't plan to post about RSD this month, I was just talking with a friend about the poem "A Crabby Old Man" (posted by Liz Hall). In the discussion with my friend, Shirley, she broke down in tears saying she couldn't continue reading Liz's observation that people don't really "see us"...admitting that she misses the old me and she mourns for both of us the busyness and vibrancy that was lost too soon and the plans of us enjoying old age together. My response was to try and console this loved one that although those things were in fact lost to me and I, too, mourn them, my consolation is that I now have an added dimension to my life. Though hard to explain or even grasp, I used the analogy that as a baby grows to adulthood and then to old age, things in adulthood are missed but old age is not without blessings. In old age, you may be lacking abilities, vigor and vibrancy but those things may be replaced with other significant qualities and activities. In my case, the "alternate life" holds crafting, writing and a drive to make a difference...and truth be told, the able-bodied Jane was responsible and fun-loving but not intent on making a difference in life. Now, however, it consumes me. My main purpose used to be raising a family and sharing the Gospel. Now there's an added dimension of ministering to hurting people and making a difference in the cause of RSD. Though I would not choose this lifestyle, I can't deny that I'm better for it.

# 2011-The Year In Review

Though I'm writing this a little bit late, it's only fitting to ring out the old and ring in the new. I don't want to say that 2011 was a bad year, but it was a hard year for me due to worsening health. On top of that, I was plagued with computer problems most of the year and I lost a couple of dear friends, which breaks my heart. But, on the flip side, I got a new grandson and some family members came for a visit from overseas. I wrote/produced a song about RSD and was blessed in many ways throughout the year. The RSD community reached new heights in 2011 through the dedication of so many who tirelessly employed their gifts and abilities. Now it is a new year with new experiences and new opportunities, new challenges and avenues for growth. I think awareness of RSD was raised significantly in 2011 and will continue doing so with increased momentum. We can't and won't stop until a cure is found. My prayer for us all in 2012 is:

May the Lord make His face to shine upon us
May He answer all our prayers
May He lead us in triumphal procession
When on Him we cast our cares

# If Given A Choice

Anyone who has read my book In the Blink of an Eye knows that I am homebound. And anyone who follows my blog knows I am now bed bound, as well. With that said, let me tell you how fiercely independent I am and why I think that's a good thing. First of all, I can't stand to be idle, and second of all, there's too much work to be done. In addition, I need to utilize my remaining abilities as long as I can. I may be confined to bed but I try to remain active to whatever degree possible…a thread that I see throughout the sick community; we're all fighting to maintain whatever abilities we have left , along with our independence. I think it's important to leave a mark on this world by giving back somehow, and writing is what I have to give. Hopefully, the legacy I leave my family will include integrity, woman of faith and crusader for change. Hence, the meaning of the title…If given a choice, I would do whatever it takes to protect my well-being and extend my usefulness.

Clearly, if I was not of sound mind, the choice would be lost, but, until then, I revel in the grace of God and respect of loved ones. Despite the commonalities, RSD affects everyone differently, and for me it holds extreme frailty, which makes ambulance rides and hospital visits way too risky. If a wrist can be permanently disabled from flipping a light switch, how much more dangerous is an ambulance ride or being pressed, pulled, prodded and moved without any warning? Knowing my body, I'm not willing to take these chances (if given a choice!).

At the start of the new year (2012), someone posed the question on Facebook "What plans do you have in the new year to improve your situation?" Because fear is one of my shortcomings and I know it's an area of my life that God is dealing with, my response was "to be braver." And, while I knew that was an apt reply, I didn't know what lie ahead or the depth of courage it would require.

On January sixth, six days into a new medicine, I became very ill and kept nothing down for the next week. Along with nausea and vomiting. I realized I was impacted from constipation. That's when I knew this was not something I ate. Rather, these were the side effects of the new drug I had started. I will not name the drug because the drug is not bad; it is, in fact, helping many people. Being hyper-sensitive to drugs, I hate trying anything new as, more often than not, the drug or the side effects will be a problem. The common side effects for this drug are constipation and nausea. Before proceeding, let me say that this subject is very personal and is only being shared in the hope of helping others. It turns out that the black liquid I was vomiting up was the contents of the small intestine due to the obstruction. I could see what it looked like but I couldn't accept that it was really happening. I went into "denial," telling myself it wasn't possible (and stayed in denial). Being unable to keep anything down, I started drinking Pedialyte to restore electrolytes, and it gave me diarrhea, which resolved the impaction and the vomiting then subsided. Later, when a friend came to help me, she told me that can happen with impaction. I called my nurse a few days later for her professional opinion and she confirmed what my friend said and felt that was exactly what had happened. Tomorrow my doctor is coming and I will see if he confirms the diagnosis, as I don't want to make any assumptions. The vomiting was so bad that I couldn't talk and, even if I could, my brain would not process such a thing…so it went unspoken. Through this whole process, my daughter was my mainstay. She feared I could die (and I knew that was possible), but she also understood that the hospital and ambulance would surely injure me. Of course I, in this frail body, could weigh the possibility of death against the certainty of injury and refuse that risk. But she, not in this body, somehow understood that calling 911 was not the solution. I cannot tell you what that meant to me. My doctor, who I thought was on vacation because he wasn't available for two weeks, was really just booked. He typically makes every effort to keep me out of the hospital, as does my nurse…partly for the risk of injury and partly for the risk of MRSA. The caregiver, however, could not see beyond normal protocol and quit the job because I wouldn't let her call 911. Earlier, I said

I kept nothing down for a week and that was literal; not water, popsicles, Pedialyte…nothing, until having a movement. Though I am no longer sick per se, it takes time to recover from that. I'm back to eating, but my stomach still feels heavy and crampy and it takes time to become regular again on your own. My daughter had scheduled a doctor appointment with a substitute but he never showed up. Finally, today, I got to see my doctor, who explained to me about vomiting up the contents of the small intestine that couldn't come out the normal way. I understand through him and Nurse Mandinec that although the small intestine contains colonic material it is different than the contents of the actual colon, as one is liquid and one would have form. In hindsight, I believe I went through a lot but also that I was spared a lot; in essence God protected me. Not only did my daughter take care of me while I was sick, she also dealt with the flood that occurred simultaneously, until my friend arrived to help. Yes, my entire apartment flooded and is now in a shambles. Ironically, I'm in the bed undisturbed, while caregivers and friends are laboring for me. What a feeling that is: gratitude, guilt, remorse (all of the above).

ServePro came in this week to assess the damage. They were scheduled last week but didn't make it till this week when my best friend was here to help, which I consider providential. My friend helped care for me and worked with the crew in moving furniture and re-locating essentials. She and another friend were a tremendous help to me. Likewise, some caregivers. Thus far, the work crew has removed all the carpet and all the baseboards and drilled holes in baseboard areas and set up fans and de-humidifiers to dry out the moisture. Fans and de-humidifiers had to be out a minimum of three days and have now been removed. And that's just the start! The work they expect to do is quite extensive. Fortunately, God is with me and His grace is sufficient. To some that may sound trite but, in reality, it's very assuring. There were so many people praying for me and, in one case, my friend sat in a chair as proxy while her church prayed healing for me. I may not know the full impact of that till I get to Heaven, but I know that kind of faith can move mountains. And I sob every time I think of such intercession for me!

Another grace/provision would be removing all the carpet without disturbing me in any way. The crew was so considerate, they never even bumped me. And, though they thought they would have to move the bed in this process, I woke up the day the work was scheduled and realized God had already provided the solution through my adjustable bed. Raising up one end at a time would accommodate removal of the carpet. And it did! (all but a 1" strip from side to side) It took a willingness on the part of the crew, but God brought it all together. At times like that, you see that He sent the provision before you even knew of the need. Though I am mortified to be so open and public about something so private, I sincerely hope it will help someone else just through being informed.

I enjoy my life, and God knows I love my family, but my becoming bed bound was caused by poor treatment of a nurse and the thought of losing more ability from rough or poor treatment is too disheartening for me. I trust God with my life and if He takes me to be with Him in Heaven that is a far greater glory than living with additional pain and limitation. I live my life to the fullest, but when my time here is up, I will be in a better place. I know that there are different beliefs, but because I believe in the saving power of Jesus Christ, I don't have to fear death. It's really that simple. In the writing of this story, I was very conflicted and actually wrote/re-wrote the story three times. At times like that, you question "Is this story not meant to be told or is it under attack for the good to be blocked?" I pray that it was in fact meant to be told and will be used for good.

Blessings,
Jane

# Depression

I don't know if blogging at this time is a good idea as I'm not really in a positive state, but there is always positive in anything if we just shift our focus. So I will endeavor to do that, to shift my focus. I feel depressed right now, for many reasons. Partly because I haven't gotten back on my meds since the sickness at the first of the year. I keep trying to but they are affecting me adversely, so I'm at a standstill, more-or-less. Also, I think I was unprepared for the progression of the disease and how encompassing it is. I think I've come to see that pain albeit horrific is just part of it. Trouble swallowing, vision loss, muscle atrophy and so much more are new dimensions to deal with. We are all capable of getting depressed, and facing these emotions head-on is actually healthy/therapeutic, but staying in the depression is not healthy. I see such despair in the pain community right now, much more than usual. And I'm here to ask that we would be earnestly praying for each other. I know that I fare better when I look at the Lord instead of the circumstance. I pray for all of us that "when you walk through the fire you will not be burned." Isaiah 43:2 NIV.

Love to all who are fighting this battle.

Jane G.

# Newness

In my last post about two weeks ago, I was dealing with depression of my own and seeing so much sorrow throughout the RSD community as well. Since that time, I have felt your prayers and support take the edge off my own circumstance and I have also seen some new and good things happening within the RSD community, things like the 2nd Annual Hope Over Pain CRPS/RSD Awareness & Research Cookbook get underway, the creation of an RSD comic book, the creation of a magazine, the one-year anniversary of Joseph Aquilino's blogtalkradio shows and other awareness projects. To make a play on words, this gives me "hope over pain." Thanks for all your prayers and support. May we all experience grace in our circumstance. God bless.

# A Battle

To those of you who read this blog, I hope today's post will speak to you somehow, that you could relate to it and feel less alone or less discouraged. This post is not about anything profound, just perspective of life with chronic illness. It's not a "how-to" or a solution. It's just a personal study of where I am in the RSD marathon. For those who have read my last two posts, you know the most current challenge has been depression. What, for me, used to be vent, re-focus and keep busy....suddenly became a fight that had me "down for the count." Because my depression came from the loss of meds I had been on and because I don't do well with meds, in general, I don't want to experiment with new ones. Being tenacious, I would rather continue my attempts at re-acclimating myself to the former drugs, little by little, till I can again tolerate them...or maybe, God forbid, go without. For now, I have learned that this is a battle, and I have discovered some weapons of warfare. I listen to music more now, I watch funnier movies, I've re-connected with poetry, I now belong to a support group and I pray even more than before. In addition to all that, I cut my hair and resumed wearing lipstick...lol. These things, no matter how small or silly, are helping. I may not be where I want to be but I'm moving forward, and that's what counts. I know that some people have major depression that requires medicine and more, and my heart goes out to you, but the point I'm making is that this is a battle and we need to be armed.

Love, Jane

# Muscles and Medicare

As many of you know, I have been bed bound for sixteen months now. Initially, I was confined to bed with severe leg ulcers but, after two months, the muscles in my shoulder and hip atrophied…which then prevented me from getting up thereafter. Since then, my doctor and I have repeatedly tried to get (soft tissue) massage therapy and mild PT to slow down ensuing debilitation. Despite trying different nursing agencies, the answer remained the same; Medicare will not pay for it unless it will enable me to walk. That is their guideline, their "measurable goal," and they need assurance of that outcome before covering the treatment/service. As the patient, my objective/"measurable goal" is to maintain movement in bed and slow down further debilitation.

Please understand that for twenty-six years I pushed myself to keep going and retain mobility through pain and limitations. It stands to reason I would continue that pursuit, albeit a lesser degree of mobility. I know the ramifications of immobility and wanted to circumvent those ramifications. Yet, without Medicare coverage or funds of my own, my hands were tied and the obvious has happened. I am now experiencing widespread atrophy of my muscles and tissue. I see my body wasting away before my very eyes. I don't know how to express my dismay at this outcome or at the flaws in the system. Though I could well be called a crusader, I am not a revolutionary or activist. I am not able to speak before the Senate. I am, though, able to raise awareness by telling my story in conjunction with everyone else's story and hope that eventually change will come.

# Clarity

I know I've not been diligent with the blog in this new year and would like to explain why. It isn't that I've lost interest or become lazy. Rather, I am at a critical place with the muscle atrophy and writing has become a struggle for me as it's hard to write with a focus on the positive while you're grieving. Awareness will always be a priority to me, which is why I keep telling my story. We all have a story and, if we share it, others are helped by it and still others are educated by it. Though I had future plans of making this into a book, I now feel a rush to complete so many things while I can still type, like this and the poetry book, etc. If what we go through can help others, it is not in vain. Thank you for your support, and God bless!

# Update

I can't believe it's been six weeks since I last posted. A lot has happened since then, the main thing being that the grieving has stopped. I can't explain that, because the situation is essentially still grievous. Yet, somehow, I've come to terms with it and actually consider this post to be full of good news. First of all, I have finished several projects that were important to me, some for awareness and some for posterity. Secondly, I am now getting (gentle) massage therapy through a means other than Medicare. Obviously, I am thrilled about that. It's beneficial in the sense that it keeps me limber, which has allowed me to maintain bed mobility. Although I can't tell you the atrophy has stopped, I can tell you that some of it is noticeably smaller. Yes, I recognize that is a miracle and I hope it continues. I hope you can appreciate the tightrope/balancing act of seeing the bad, yet focusing on the good, praying and rejoicing with me. May the stories we share and events we hold expedite public awareness, and may our prayers for each other have great effect. Blessings, Jane

# A birthday post from an aged RSD'er...lol !

As of today, I am officially "OLD"!...and, strange as it seems, I am thrilled! There's no more dread of getting old, no more sweating the small stuff, not as many insecurities and a lot more comfort in your own skin. I love the person I've become and appreciate the people who made the journey with me.

All too often, we perceive aging as a lessening when, in fact, it's an increase. It's the sum of wisdom and knowledge you've acquired, it's the heightened respect and the decreased rebellion. It is sometimes a slower pace with added purpose. It is often a keener sense and clearer vision. It is, basically, expansion, which is more, not less.

What does this have to do with RSD, you ask! As an RSD'er of twenty-seven years, it's proof that we can cope and survive all that illness throws at us. We can live a full life albeit painful. I am grateful to God for this stage of life and for all He's brought me through. I consider myself very blessed and all of you are part of the blessing.

Love,
Jane

# Sufficient Grace

"Sometimes God calms the storm...sometimes He lets the storm rage and calms His child." I don't know who said that, but it's certainly true. Blogging has been somewhat of a challenge for me in 2012 due to added health issues, sometimes because the pain is so bad and sometimes because you can't find the words to articulate the pros and cons, good and bad, peace and frustration of your life. I stand in amazement that God's grace is sufficient, but all you RSD'ers out there know that doesn't equate to easy. Even bearable is debatable. See why it's hard to articulate. You're grateful to wake up each day to an everlasting love and tender mercies, but the pain seems so unbearable. I have to keep reminding myself that everyone has something, be it a broken body or a broken heart.

I won't go into the added health issues because it would make the post too "heavy." On the bright side, my poetry book is in production and this book has been approved for publication, I'm still able to type and craft, I have friends, family and good care. What more can I say?

You are all in my prayers. I wish you abundant blessings and minimal pain.

Love,
Jane

# Back In The Saddle Again

After months of agonizing pain, I finally feel somewhat decent (by RSD standards, that is). I know the regular pain and symptoms we deal with are bad enough but flares and added issues can put our pain levels over the top. Fortunately, some med changes were helpful in bringing things under control. Yet, I'm always amazed at the number of secondary issues that come with RSD, or the side effects from meds, or complications from a procedure. So with all of that going on, it is comforting to have the prayers, wishes and overall support from each other. I'm surely not glad to have RSD but I'm glad to know the compassion and kindness of so many in this community.

In closing, mine is a story of what can happen, not necessarily what will happen. Everyone's story is different. Some cases seem better off, while others seem worse off. Whichever the case…though RSD affects your body, don't let it affect your spirit. Cling to the grace of God and cherish the blessings in your life. By making the most of each day, you will be better for it.

# Afterword

Having dealt with RSD alone for so many years, I would encourage everyone with RSD to partake of the mentoring program offered through RSD Hope. It is a partnership with someone who understands and relates to what you're going through. It is a give and take: a learning, teaching, growing experience and a blessing beyond measure.